# 6 Pack After 60

A Simple & Effective System

For Getting & Staying Strong

By James E. Hess

James E. Hess Publications

4417 13th Street, St. Cloud, FL. 34769, USA

http://www.6PackAfter60.com

Cover photo and illustrations by Rebecca Cotton-Hess

# Disclaimer

You are advised to get your physician's approval before beginning this exercise program. The recommendations are not medical guidelines but are for educational purposes only.

You should consult your physician prior to starting this program or if you have any medical condition or injury. This program is designed for healthy individuals 18 years and older only.

It is strongly recommended that you have a complete physical examination if you are sedentary, have high cholesterol, high blood pressure, or diabetes, or you are overweight.

If you experience any lightheadedness, dizziness, or shortness of breath while exercising, stop the movement and consult a physician.

All forms of exercise pose some inherent risks. The author and publisher advise readers to take full responsibility for their safety and know their limits. The author and publisher are not liable for any injuries incurred while following this program. The exercises in this program are not intended as a substitute for any exercise routine or treatment that may have been prescribed by your physician.

## Dedication

*To my wife and best friend, Becky, for your belief and trust in me for many years.*

*Also to my boys, Jared and Jaxon, you guys make me feel like a kid again.*

# Contents

# Introduction

Sometime after I turned 55, my wife Becky and I adopted two infant boys. We had been their foster parents since birth. I knew if I was going to be able to keep up with them as they got older, I needed to do something that would keep me strong and would not take much time.

I have wasted so much time and effort trying to get in shape and stay in shape...........but you won't.

If you're looking for the fastest, and most effective way to get stronger and physically fit, you found it.

This book will change your life for the better. It will also save you a lot of time, effort, and money getting and staying physically fit.

Just about anyone can benefit from this SYSTEM.. Whether you are a teenager or many years older than myself, you will get stronger. Don't let the title mislead you. A six pack is nice to have, but it is far from the focus of this book.

If you have never exercised or it has been awhile, there is a starting point that will fit you.

If you are in excellent shape, this will challenge you.

I would suggest you read this like a book. Begin at chapter one and don't jump around. Please resist the temptation to start with the exercise chapters.

The effectiveness of this program is the SYSTEM. By reading from the beginning you will understand its importance for your success, and most importantly, your staying with the program.

# Chapter One

# My Story

Since my first introduction to weight training at age 9, I was semi-obsessed with getting stronger. I don't think I was too different than any other kid back then or kids today. With the vast assortment of super heroes today, being strong is definitely in vogue.

As strange as this seems, I can still remember the older kids in the neighborhood, who were probably 13 or 14 years old at the time, recruiting me and my friend to be their weight training experiments. I'm sure we didn't do much heavy lifting back then, but it definitely kick-started my journey to where I am today and why I wrote this book.

I have been experimenting since that day with various methods of strength training, so it could arguably be stated that I have around 50 years experience in what does and doesn't work. How many people do you know who have fifty years of experience in ANYTHING, and are still alive?

In high school, I was given a set of weights by my cousin. He never used them. Very typical, most weight sets never get used much if at all. But I really used mine. A good friend at the time, Charlie, used to come to my house on Saturday mornings to work out. The weights were kept in our basement. My grandfather made a wooden bench (at my request) to be used to do bench presses.

I remember the day Charlie was spotting (hovering over the weights in case I couldn't press it all the way up) me when the bench broke. First one side of the barbell dumped the weights on the floor then immediately the same for the other side. I didn't get hurt but the basement tile did.

## College Days

In college at the University of Cincinnati, I joined the power lifting team. Everything was centered on just three lifts: Bench Press, Dead Lift, and Squat.

These movements are all about strength and technique. I got into it for a while until I started noticing the best lifters. They had huge thighs, big hips, big butts, and big guts.

But they could lift a lot of iron. I didn't want to look like them. I liked the way the body builders looked so I switched.

Then I started on those long marathon workouts that lasted 2 hours or more. Needing to get in all those sets for each body part took time. What a waste of effort and time. I was very fortunate that I didn't injure myself.

Sometime during my college years, a new exercise system came on the scene. It was called Nautilus. This was a combination of different machines that worked different body parts. Each machine was referred to as a station. When you went through all the stations, that was a complete workout cycle.

If you were in really good shape you could go through two cycles. In great shape, go through 3 cycles. The faster you could go through the cycle (less rest in between the stations) was an indication of your physical fitness.

I did the Nautilus routine for a year or so but eventually went back to lifting weights.

## After College

Throughout the years after college, it became harder and harder to "hit the gym" and "get a good workout in."

I eventually moved my gym equipment inside my home. Using a combination of different machines along with free weights I was able to get more consistent workouts.

As I was approaching the age of 50, I noticed that I was taking a lot of time off because of injuries, especially lower back.

One Saturday morning I was doing some dumbbell squats, lowering myself almost to the floor while holding two very heavy (at least for me) 65 lb. dumbbells. Since I was feeling so good, I decided to pump out a few extra reps. That's when I heard a loud popping sound in my lower back. After falling to the ground I could barely crawl to the couch in the family room.

Three or four days of lying around and putting up with intense spasms, I had to rethink my routine. Clearly my current training methods did not have longevity.

Around that time my wife and I decided to be foster parents. It was really Becky's idea and I just went along with it. We started taking in drug-exposed babies. This left even less time now to get a good, consistent workout.

In hindsight, this was a good thing, and not just for the babies we took in.
It forced me to come up with a system that was not only sustainable, but effective and flexible.

In 2007 another major event in my life forced me to come up with the System that I have today.

At that time we did not have a foster child living with us. Then we got the call. A two day old baby boy (born at the hospital down the street) was in need of a home. We took him. We were prepared with a crib and all the necessary paraphernalia since we had just fostered another baby a few months earlier that went back to her mother.

Then another baby boy was born two days later at the same hospital. A few months later we were asked to take him. We did.

I know you have to be thinking, "what has this to do with a book about a fitness system?" Everything! Let me finish.

So, now my wife, Becky and I have two infant baby boys living with us. I forgot to mention that we had Becky's parents move in with us a year earlier after her Dad was diagnosed with terminal cancer. Also we both had demanding full time jobs at the time. I know it sounds like I'm making this up but it's all true.

But wait, it gets even more exciting.

In 2008, we were informed by the case workers that both babies were going up for adoption. One of the mothers voluntarily terminated her rights and the other mother just disappeared. Her rights were terminated by a judge. So, we adopted both boys, within 90 days of each other, before they turned one. This was a few months after I turned 56.

Now to bring you to the present.

We are in the Fall of 2012 and the boys, Jared and Jaxon are 5 years old and just started Kindergarten.

I am 60 years old. Oh yeah, I also have a 6 pack!!! The System works.

# Chapter Two

# A National Epidemic

Hardly a week goes by that you don't see a newspaper headline or magazine article about America's obesity crisis.

First of all, let's define obesity. According to medical websites, a person is obese if they are more than 20% over their ideal weight.

## *What is an ideal weight?*

It depends on your height, age, sex, and build.
According to the BMI (Body Mass Index) everyone has an ideal weight range based on height and age.

If you want to check yours, go to www.bmi-calculator.net.

This is a fairly accurate indicator to show if you are overweight. However, this is not a fail-safe measurement. It does not distinguish between fat and muscle.
Because of this minor flaw, a very muscular NFL linebacker would probably be overweight and maybe even obese using this index. But, for most of us, this is accurate.

So, since the obesity rate is currently 36% of all Americans and is projected to be 42% by 2030, I would say this is a major problem. The most tragic part of this problem is the children who are obese. Children being obese was almost unheard of a few generations ago.

Now, if obesity is traditionally defined as being 20% or more over one's ideal weight, what about all the people who are 10% or 15% over their ideal weight?

They are just classified as overweight. What percentage do you think this would be? I wouldn't be surprised if all Americans classified as obese and overweight would be 90% or more.

Now this is the funny part. The reality is that approximately 6 out of every 10 Americans are overweight. Yet in surveys taken, only 4 out of 10 perceive themselves to be overweight. Talk about denial. This is where the BMI can inject a little reality into some people.

## Being overweight can be expensive.

The cost estimates of treating obesity-related conditions run over $150 billion a year. Obese and even overweight people are at a higher risk for a variety of ailments. Some of these are diabetes, heart disease, stroke, osteoarthritis, acid reflux, early dementia, reproductive problems, and up to nine types of cancer.

The majority of this cost is passed on to us in the form of higher insurance premiums and government programs.

The less we exercise, the fatter (as a nation) we get, the more we all have to pay. Right now this payment averages about $1,500 per household and appears to be heading upward. Think of this as an annual tax.

Just what we all need, another tax, right.

There's no mystery why the American waistline is expanding. Food providers are very good at giving people what they want, namely sugar, salt and fat. If you have ever tasted a McDonald's french fry, a potato chip, or a corn chip, you know it's very hard to stop at just one. You want to keep on eating.

Because they are in business to make a profit, providers load all three (sugar, salt, and fat) into food to give people what they want. The outcome for them is that they make a ton of money.

I need to explain something at this point.

I have no problem with the food providers making a big profit. That's why they took the risk and started the business in the first place.

I especially would not want any governmental "food police" telling me what I can and cannot eat. I'm all for personal freedom of choice, as long as we still have a choice.

The market will always give us what we want. Which means they will always give us what we are willing to pay for at a profit for the provider.

So, if we as a nation start to demand healthier choices for food consumption, the market will provide them. Fortunately this is starting to happen.

Look at the more nutritious items on any of the popular fast food chains menus. They weren't there 10 years ago.

So why do we still have a national weight problem? That's easy. People are not making the right food choices, eating too much, and not exercising enough or at all.

I'll be offering more in depth solutions for eating better in my next book which will be focused on food.

The title will be "The 6 Pack After 60 No-Diet Diet". Hope you will read it. It will change your life. In fact, it might even save your life.

# Chapter Three

# Introducing the PSP Fitness System

Before I explain the basics, you need to know why it's called a system.

## *What is a system?*

One of the definitions is:  a set of interacting or interdependent components forming an integrated whole.

Let me give you an illustration.  Have you ever eaten a McDonald's hamburger?  (You could substitute Burger King, Wendy's, etc.).

Do you think, even if you aren't much of a cook, that you could make a better tasting burger than a McDonald's hamburger?  Of course you could, I know I could.  In fact I have done so numerous times.

But, there's always a "but."  Could you make your better tasting burger "consistently" for around 68 million customers every day in 119 countries like McDonald's does?  Not without a system that McDonald's has perfected.

Let me give you another analogy.  Everyone would probably agree that it's good to brush your teeth (at least once in awhile).  Also most people would agree that flossing your teeth is a good idea.  Let's not forget a visit to the dentist, especially if there is a problem.  All three of these things are good to do.

But when and how often?  Hit or miss or a purposeful system?

How about brushing and flossing your teeth twice each day, mornings and evenings, every day.  Combine that with an every six months visit to the dentist for a cleaning and checkup with x-rays taken once a year.

That's a dental hygiene system I've been following for decades.  It has served me well since I haven't had even a minor issue in over 15 years.

So to give you the basics of the PSP Fitness System;

There are only 3 basic types of movements needed: Push, Squat, and Pull.

I say basic because there are many different variations within these three compound movements, but all the variations work the same muscle groups as the basic.

# Compound vs. Isolation Exercises

Isolation exercises work only one muscle at a time. Some examples of these would be a dumbbell curl (bicep) or a one-legged calf raise. These exercises are very time consuming, inefficient, and can lead to injuries if not experienced and warmed-up sufficiently.

Compound exercises work many muscles and muscle groups simultaneously. Also they simulate real-world activities. You burn more calories while you improve coordination, joint stability, reaction time and balance.

A Push exercise uses muscles in the chest, shoulders, triceps, forearms, back and abdominals.

A Pull exercise uses back, biceps, shoulders, forearms and abdominals.

A Squat exercise uses hips, lower back, thighs, calves, and abdominals.

Notice that all three work the abdominals (stomach), so sit-ups, crunches, or any other type of abdominal exercise is never needed.

One part of the System is the variations of the Push, Squat, and Pulling movements, such as repetitions, sets, frequency, etc.

# Importance of a Log

Another main component of the System is keeping a log (see Resources section). There are only two; a weekly (to record your daily activity), and a monthly log (to give you a bigger picture of your improvement)

Included within the weekly log is a place to record your weight and waistline measurement. This is critical to your success!!!

Plan on weighing yourself and measuring your waistline (get a simple tape measure) only once a week. Pick a certain day and time and stick to it. I do mine every Sunday morning as soon as I get out of bed. (Daily weighing and measuring are a waste of time. Don't do it!)

This way you will have an accurate assessment of your improvement. This is an extremely important aspect of the System and has a positive psychological effect. This will help with your diet and with your consistency. I'll explain more about this later.

The other important part of the system is your picture. With cameras in just about every phone, this is a very easy task. Take your picture from the knees up and if possible have someone take it from behind. You should be wearing a bathing suit or something similar. You want as much skin exposed as possible.
Date these pictures and repeat every three to four months ( just 3 or 4 times a year).

This will be a gigantic motivator when you can start to see the positive changes in your body. In fact, I'll have a blog set up for those who would like to share their progress and pictures with others. Your pictures just might inspire someone to get started.

## System Summary

- The 3 basic movements

- The weekly log of what you did and when you did it

- Your weight and waistline weekly measurements

- Your quarterly front and back pictures

**The only thing left is to start and don't stop**.

I'll get into more details about how and when to start in a later chapter.

# Chapter Four

## Milo of Croton

I included this character to illustrate a principle.

Milo was an extremely athletic wrestler around the 6th century BC.   Ancient Greeks were very into their games or competitive events, just like the Olympics today.

Milo was known for his extraordinary strength.
He was said to have carried an ox on his shoulders through the stadium at Olympia.   That surely got the crowd on their feet.

During his wrestling career, he won 32 competitions, was a six time Olympic victor, and won seven crowns at the Pythian Games at Delphi.  His competitive career spanned a quarter of a century.

He died (see  picture) when he was attempting to tear a tree apart and his hands became trapped in the the cleft of its trunk.  This didn't kill him but left him semi-defenseless when a pack of wolves surprised and devoured him.

Hard to believe that story.  I'm glad there was a picture to back it up.

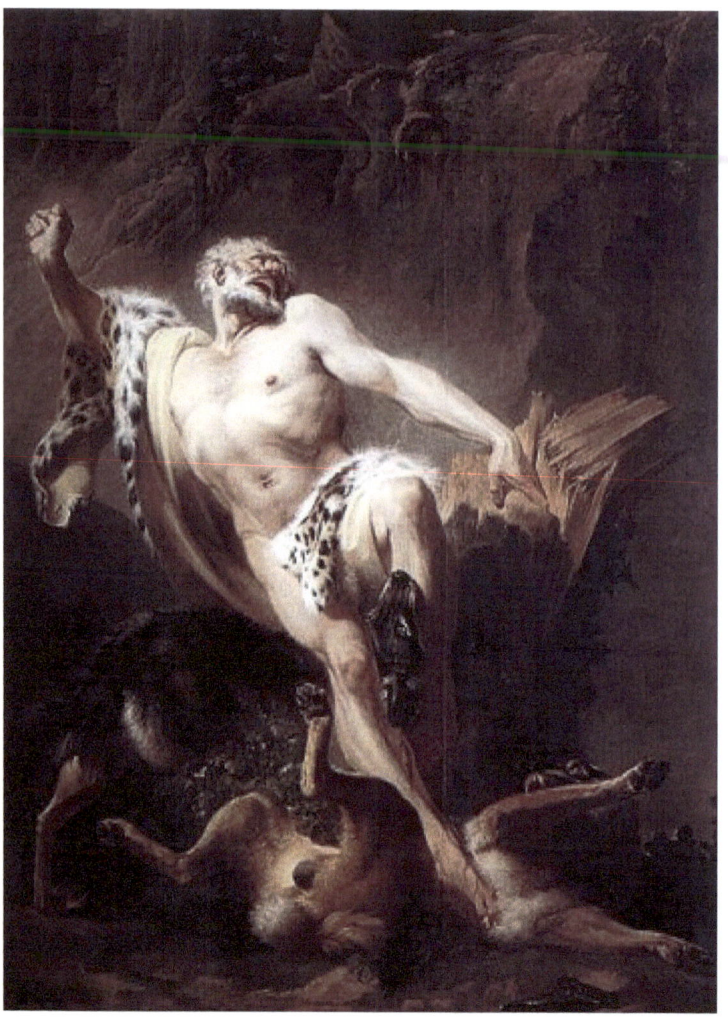

**What Was His Secret?**

How did this guy train to get so strong and stay strong for so long (at least until the wolves got him)? Even in the picture you can tell he was fairly old by the white hair and beard. But look at the shape he was in!

According to his legend, he trained by carrying a calf daily from its birth until it became a full-sized ox. That was why he was able to carry that ox around the stadium whenever the urge hit him.

Seriously, here is the principle. He exercised every day, lifting progressively more weight each day as the calf got bigger.

I'm advocating that you exercise every day, or at least five or six days every week.

You won't need to lift more weight each week, because you won't be lifting anything but yourself. You will start doing more repetitions of each exercise because you will get stronger.

This will be very gradual, that's why you log everything you do, every day you do it. Also, when you start to do 2 to 3 times more repetitions (of any given movement) than when you started, it will be with less effort than when you began. Why? Because you will be much stronger and in better condition.

Milo's training method is a great example of a sustainable system. Obviously, only for him.

# Chapter Five

# Me & Arnold

Arnold Schwarzenegger was born July 30, 1947. He began to weight train at the age of 15. He was Mr. Universe at age 20 and went on to win the Mr. Olympia contest seven times.

Posters of him were in gyms around the world in the 1970s. He looked unbelievable. We all wanted to look like Arnold.

His workouts were legendary. Sometimes he would perform two workouts per day. He had books about his work-outs; supposedly his exact training routine.

I'm sure many guys tried to follow it in hopes of looking like him. The routines were just about impossible to do for any length of time. Way too many hours in the gym.

Today, if you Google "Fat Arnold" you'll see some very unflattering pictures and videos of an out of shape 50 something guy.

I don't know what kind of shape he is in now that he's in his mid 60s, probably not too good. My point in all this is not to disparage Arnold in any way. He is a phenomenal individual, successful in many ways.

I just wanted to point out that his "system" for getting strong was far from sustainable. It was only good for a short season of his life.

My younger brother, Jack, on the other hand, has a sustainable system. He is 58 years old and a CFO in the Denver, Colorado area. He played college football, on a scholarship, for the University of Cincinnati Bearcats. This is also my alma mater.

Jack still works out nearly every day since he graduated college over 36 years ago.
His only physical differences today are that he is a little stronger and a little leaner than when he played football. A consistent, sustainable system can prolong youthful physical abilities for decades.

If you used to be in great or good shape at one time in your life, what happened?

I'll tell you what happened. Whatever you did to get in great or good shape was not sustainable.

This System that I will show you is very sustainable. This is the key to noticeable results.

When I was in high school I was very athletic. I remember a time when we were given a physical fitness test. We had to climb a rope, do maximum repetitions of sit-ups and push-ups, and a few other things that I can't remember.
I do remember the push-ups because I had one of the highest scores in my class. I did 33 consecutive push-ups without a rest.

Today, over 44 years later, I do sets of 35 push-ups (with a max of 50) at least three times a week.

**This system works!!!**

# Chapter Six

## The Real Fountain of Youth

There is a common desire in most human beings to stay young when we feel our youth slipping away. Throughout history there have been stories of people searching for ways to regain their youth or at least their youthful vitality.

One of the most familiar is about Ponce de Leon and his search for the fountain of youth.

Ponce de Leon was the first Spanish explorer, or conquistador, to arrive in Florida, by way of St. Augustine. He had heard of a mythical fountain of youth from the local Indians. They spoke of a legendary, magical spring whose water was believed to make older people young again. How young? They didn't specify, just younger.

To make a very long story very short, he explored most of Florida and even the Bahamas. He never found the fountain. But he did discover Florida. That's got to count for something.

## Human Growth Hormone

I couldn't leave this one out of a chapter about the Fountain of Youth.

Human Growth Hormone, abbreviated HGH, is a protein produced by the pituitary gland. This gland is located at the base of the brain. The protein contains over 190 separate amino acids which are responsible for the growth and health of all cells in the body.

This is very potent and powerful stuff.  Here is the problem.

The rate of HGH production in the body is higher when we are young and starts decreasing as we age.
Because of this production decrease we start seeing and experiencing the signs of aging such as loss of muscle mass (we get weaker), wrinkles, hair loss, loose skin, decreased mental awareness as well as decreased libido.

This is very tough for some men to handle.  That's why middle-aged men buy convertibles, start wearing gold chains and date younger women.  Seriously, no one really wants to get old.

In 1985 synthetic human growth hormone was developed and approved by the FDA for specific uses in children and adults.  In children it is mainly used in treating genetic disorders affecting growth.  In adults it is mainly used for treating muscle-wasting diseases associated with AIDS.

Some people use the hormone to build muscle and improve athletic performance. Usually other performance-enhancing drugs such as anabolic steroids are used as well.  The effect on athletic performance using HGH is unknown.  Also it is not FDA-approved for this use.

There are many products that claim to increase your body's own production of HGH.  The companies that market these products claim they can turn back your body's biological clock, build muscle, reduce fat, restore hair growth and color, strengthen the immune system, normalize blood sugar, improve sex life, increase energy, sleep quality, vision, and memory.

Who wouldn't buy this stuff if it worked?  I certainly would!

Unfortunately there is no reliable evidence to support the claim that these products have the same effects as prescription HGH, according to the Federal Trade Commission.

The problem is that these marketed products are usually sold in the form of pills and sprays. Prescription HGH is always given by injection. Taken orally, HGH is digested by the stomach before it can be absorbed into the body.

The only good news out of all this is if you can get some pharmaceutical grade HGH and you don't mind injecting yourself every day, at a set time, without fail, you might be able to see some of those claims listed above. Of course this comes at a cost of around $1,000 a month for life. You can't stop or you'll lose all the positive efforts. Plus there are some possible side effects.

Why is there always a catch when something seems too good to be true?

Some of those side effects include high cholesterol levels, carpal tunnel syndrome, numbness and tingling of the skin, increase in the risk of diabetes, swelling due to fluid in the body's tissues, joint pain, and possible growth of cancerous tumors.

There has got to be an easier and safer way to look and feel younger and stronger.

Fortunately there is..............

Here is the only true and lasting Fountain of Youth:

## DIET AND EXERCISE

Now what kind of diet and what kind of exercise?

I'll deal specifically with the diet in my next book. For now the focus will be on the exercise part of the Youth Fountain.

# Chapter Seven

## Is There A Future In It?

This is a great question to ask yourself whenever starting something:

- When you interview for a job

- When you look to buy a house

- When you want to start a business

- When you are dating someone

- When you decide to marry

So why wouldn't you ask the question before starting an exercise program?

There is nothing wrong with trying out something new.  Check out a local gym, a piece of equipment for your home, set of weights, etc.

But, before you commit your time, effort, and money...ask the question.

Will you be using that equipment a month from now, a year from now?

Will you be working out faithfully, at least 3 to 4 times a week, at that gym for the entirety of your annual membership?  If so, great, but what about the next year, and the next?  What about the next 10 or 20 years?

The key word is sustainability.  Is your program sustainable?

# Chapter Eight

# Don't Make It An Event

This might seem like a minor issue or even a non-issue. But it is important enough to make it a separate chapter.

First, what do I mean by Don't Make It An Event? A workout or exercise session is usually something that takes some effort to prepare for, get dressed for, and probably even drive to.

For example, if you work-out at a local gym you have to prepare. You get your gym bag ready if you plan to change and shower there.

If not, you still need to get dressed in your workout attire, drive to the location, park your car, walk to the building, sign in at the front desk, then start looking for an open machine to start your exercise routine.

After finishing, you get back in your car, drive home, change your clothes, and take a shower (if you didn't pack a gym bag and shower there).

I know the routine. I did it for many years. Sometimes I got in a good work-out, sometimes I didn't, depending on how crowded the gym was that day. There was definitely no consistency.

Bottom line is that this is a very unsustainable "system" to get stronger and "stay in shape."

My system is about as eventful as showering and bushing your teeth. It is just something you do most mornings, afternoons, or evenings (depending on what works best for you) for about 5 minutes to 30 minutes, depending on your physical condition.

**IF IT ISN'T SIMPLE, EASY, AND REWARDING... IT ISN'T SUSTAINABLE.**

Doesn't a lot of your existing everyday habits fall into this category? Habits such as showering, bushing teeth, getting dressed, and eating.

# Chapter Nine

## The Importance of Logs, Measurements, and Pictures

This is equally important as the exercise movements in the next few chapters. This is the secret for you continuing with the program.

### First the logs

Here are some examples of weekly logs for three different people:

## Weekly PSP System Log

**October**

| Date | Day | Movement | Set 1 | Set 2 | Set 3 | Movement | Set 1 | Set 2 | Set 3 | Movement | Set 1 | Set 2 | Set 3 |
|------|-----|----------|-------|-------|-------|----------|-------|-------|-------|----------|-------|-------|-------|
| 1 | Mon | Push | 4 | 5 | 5 | Squat | | | | Pull | | | |
| 2 | Tues | Push | | | | Squat | 12 | 15 | 15 | Pull | | | |
| 3 | Wed | Push | | | | Squat | | | | Pull | 2 | 1 | 1 |
| 4 | Thurs | Push | 5 | 6 | 5 | Squat | | | | Pull | | | |
| 5 | Fri | Push | | | | Squat | 12 | 15 | 17 | Pull | | | |
| 6 | Sat | Push | | | | Squat | | | | Pull | 2 | 2 | 1 |
| 7 | Sun | Push | | | | Squat | | | | Pull | | | |

| Totals: | | Push: | 30 |
|---------|--|-------|----|
| (for the week) | | Squat: | 86 |
| | | Pull: | 9 |

| Weight: | 210 |
|---------|-----|
| Waist: | 39.5 |

# Weekly PSP System Log

**October**

| Date | Day | Movement | Set 1 | Set 2 | Set 3 | Movement | Set 1 | Set 2 | Set 3 | Movement | Set 1 | Set 2 | Set 3 |
|------|-----|----------|-------|-------|-------|----------|-------|-------|-------|----------|-------|-------|-------|
| 1 | Mon | Push | 8 | 10 | | Squat | 20 | 22 | | Pull | 3 | 3 | |
| 2 | Tues | Push | 8 | 8 | | Squat | 12 | 20 | | Pull | 2 | 3 | |
| 3 | Wed | Push | | | | Squat | | | | Pull | | | |
| 4 | Thurs | Push | 8 | 9 | 9 | Squat | 15 | 15 | 20 | Pull | 2 | 4 | 3 |
| 5 | Fri | Push | 8 | 10 | 9 | Squat | 12 | 15 | 17 | Pull | 3 | 2 | 3 |
| 6 | Sat | Push | | | | Squat | | | | Pull | | | |
| 7 | Sun | Push | 8 | 10 | | Squat | 15 | 17 | | Pull | 4 | 3 | |

**Totals:**

(for the week)

| | |
|---|---|
| **Push:** | 105 |
| **Squat:** | 200 |
| **Pull:** | 35 |

| | |
|---|---|
| Weight: | 135 |
| Waist: | 33 |

# Weekly PSP System Log

October

| Date | Day | Movement | Set 1 | Set 2 | Set 3 | Movement | Set 1 | Set 2 | Set 3 | Movement | Set 1 | Set 2 | Set 3 |
|------|-----|----------|-------|-------|-------|----------|-------|-------|-------|----------|-------|-------|-------|
| 1 | Mon | Push | | | | Squat | 25 | 25 | 35 | Pull | | | |
| 2 | Tues | Push | 14+18 | 15+12 | 18 | Squat | | | | Pull | 6+6 | 5 | 6 |
| 3 | Wed | Push | | | | Squat | 25+20 | 25 | 25 | Pull | | | |
| 4 | Thurs | Push | 15+16 | 15+17 | 19 | Squat | | | | Pull | 5+6 | 5+5 | 6 |
| 5 | Fri | Push | | | | Squat | 12 | 15 | 17 | Pull | | | |
| 6 | Sat | Push | 19 | 19 | | Squat | | | | Pull | 6+7 | 6 | 5 |
| 7 | Sun | Push | | | | Squat | 25+20 | 20+25 | 25 | Pull | | | |

Totals:

(for the week)

| Push: | 197 |
|-------|-----|
| Squat: | 339 |
| Pull: | 74 |

| Weight: | 187.5 |
|---------|-------|
| Waist: | 36.5 |

I want to show you the flexibility of this system. You can create a new workout routine every week if so desired. I don't recommend switching that frequently.

Every 4 to 6 weeks it is advisable to change the routine.

Here is an example of a monthly log. This gives a bigger picture of your progress:

## Monthly PSP System Log

| | Jan | Feb | March | April | May | June | July | Aug | Sept | Oct | Nov | Dec | Total |
|---|---|---|---|---|---|---|---|---|---|---|---|---|---|
| Push-Ups | 224 | 247 | 307 | 332 | 358 | 367 | | | | | | | |
| Squats | 409 | 443 | 456 | 501 | 556 | 580 | | | | | | | |
| Pull-ups | 115 | 119 | 127 | 144 | 169 | 180 | | | | | | | |
| **Beginning** | | | | | | | | | | | | | |
| Weight: | 198 | 195 | 189 | 186 | 183.5 | 181 | 179 | | | | | | |
| Waist: | 39.5 | 39 | 38.25 | 38 | 37.5 | 36.75 | 35.5 | | | | | | |
| **Ending** | | | | | | | | | | | | | |
| Weight: | 195 | 189 | 186 | 183.5 | 181 | 179 | | | | | | | |
| Waist: | 39 | 38.25 | 38 | 37.5 | 36.75 | 35.5 | | | | | | | |

## Now for the measurements

There is an old saying that has always stuck with me:

## WHATEVER IS MEASURED IMPROVES

That says it all.

A great benefit of measuring yourself weekly is that you will want to see an improvement every week. To get this improvement you will start being more conscious of everything you eat, how much you eat, and when you eat.

## Now for the pictures

This is more of a visual, psychological motivator. I recommend taking pictures of yourself in your bathing suit, front and back if possible. Remember, no one needs to see these pictures but you (and the person taking them).

You may or may not notice any big changes month to month, but check those pictures with a 3 to 4 month time frame. Those will be extremely motivating.

# Chapter Ten

## Before We Get Started

I have continually emphasized the simplicity and effectiveness of this system.

**THIS SYSTEM IS NOT ABOUT GETTING A SIX PACK** (although it is possible).

It is about getting stronger in the quickest, easiest, and most sustainable way possible.

There will be a time commitment from you, but it will never be too much. If it was, it wouldn't be sustainable, right? The time commitment each day, six days a week, will be approximately 5 to 10 minutes --- that's it!

After a period of time, depending on your present condition, you can expect to max out at no more than 30 minutes a day.

Personally, I do not average 30 minutes a day yet. I may not ever. One would have to be in extraordinary condition to average 30 minutes a day with this system.

Just to give you an idea as to where I am currently with this. I can very easily do over 100 consecutive squats. I have also done 50 consecutive push-ups, and 18 consecutive pull-ups. The last two not so easily.

These numbers may or may not impress you. That is not my intention. Here is what I want you to consider:

If a 60+ year old man can do that, using this system, it has got to do something positive for you. You will get stronger.

# Chapter Eleven

# PUSH

There are so many exercises and so many ways to do them, it is no wonder that people never get started.  It can be very confusing. This system will be kept simple.

This is the first of three types of PUSH movements.  There are literary dozens of push type movements; some using weights and others using machines, bands, cables, or equipment.

There will be no more than 3 movements per each section.  You need to know that within these 3 are many different variations.  Again, to keep things simple we won't be discussing all the variations.

All these PUSH movements will primarily strengthen the chest, shoulders, triceps, back, and abdominals.  The variations in hand placement will only affect the degree of emphasis on each of the above body parts.  So, in general, don't worry about hand placement at this time.
Your main focus should be on perfecting the movement.  Keep this in mind always.

**YOU ARE NOT EXERCISING.**

**YOU ARE PRACTICING THE MOVEMENTS TO PERFECTION.**

Let's start with the PUSH.

The first movement is a bent knee push-up.
(See illustrations)

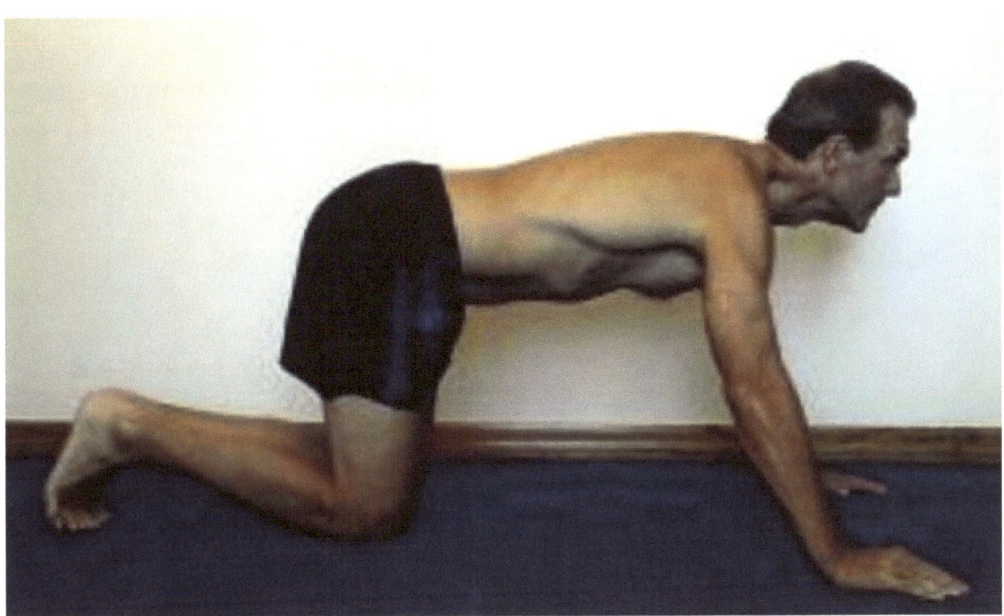

**Remember to stay focused on perfecting the movement**

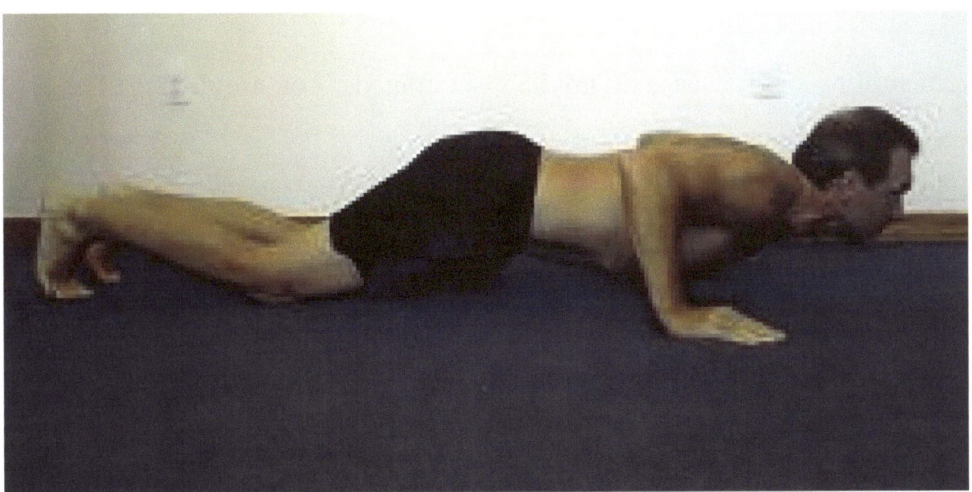

Get on the floor and position your hands slightly wider than your shoulders. The wider your hands position the more emphasis on the chest. The more narrow your hands position the more emphasis on the triceps.

Be sure to keep the knees, hips and shoulders all in a straight line. Do not bend at the hips like you are bowing, this will disengage the body parts you are trying to strengthen.

Before you begin, contract your abs and tighten your core by pulling your belly button toward your spine. Keep a tight core throughout the entire movement.

If you cannot lower yourself to the floor, just go half way or a quarter of the way.

Inhale as you slowly bend your elbows and lower yourself. Exhale as you begin pushing back up to the start position.

Do not lock your elbows at the top of the movement but continue to lower yourself again. Do this for as many repetitions as is comfortable.

When you start to lose good form, stop.
I would recommend working up to three sets. One set to start is fine.

When you are able to do 20 continuous repetitions, start on the next movement.

If you stay on this movement for months please do not be discouraged. You are getting stronger every week. Your logs will prove this to you.

The second movement is the traditional push-up.

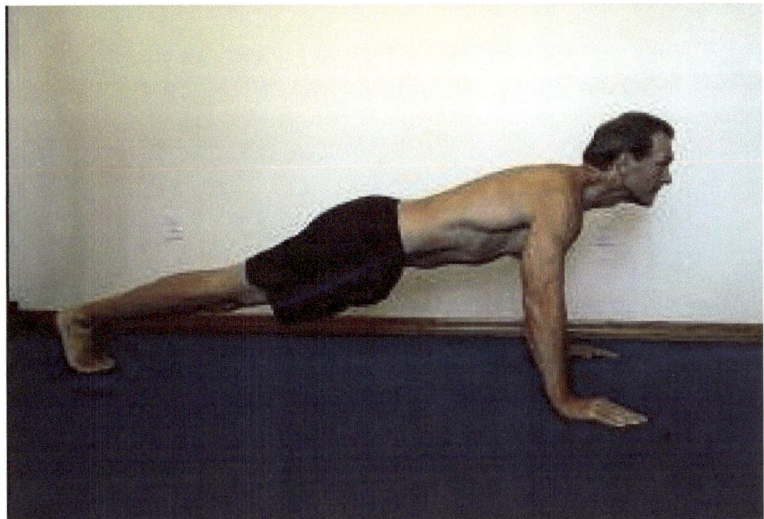

**Focus on perfecting the movement**

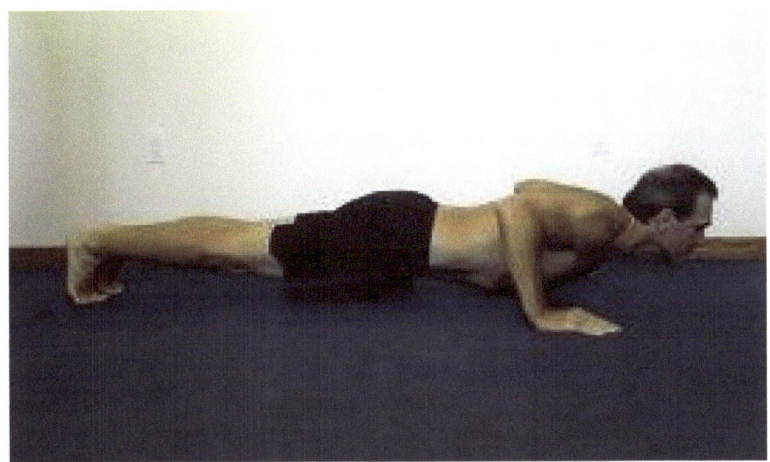

Do not advance to this movement until you are able to perform around 20 continuous repetitions of the first movement. Once you advance, you will never go back to the first movement.

The push-up has been called the perfect total body exercise that builds both upper body and core strength when done properly.

Get on the floor and position your hands slightly wider than your shoulders as in the first movement.

Raise up onto your toes so you are balanced on your hands and toes. (see illustration)

Keep your body in a straight line from head to toe without arching your back or sagging in the middle.
Your feet position may be close together or a bit wider. Get a feel for what is the most comfortable.

Contract your abdominals and tighten your core by pulling you belly button toward your spine. Work on contracting your arms and chest also throughout the entire movement.

Inhale as you slowly bend your elbows and lower yourself until your elbows are at a 90 degree angle or you have slightly touched your chest on the floor.

Keep your head up and eyes looking forward in the down position.

Exhale as you begin pushing back up to the start position.

Don't lock out the elbows; keep them slightly bent.

Repeat the movement until you start to lose form.

If you cannot do at least 3 -5 good repetitions, start back on the first movement until your strength increases.

Work up to three sets, but one good set is fine at the beginning.

The third movement is a decline push-up.  (See illustrations)

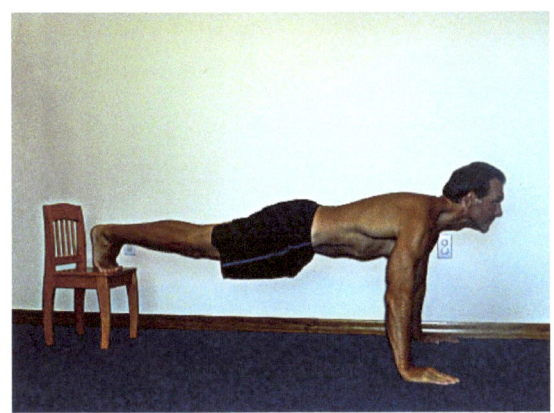

**Concentrate on breathing correctly**

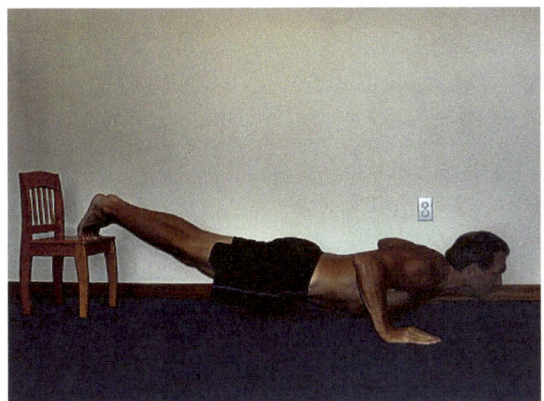

This is exactly the same as the push-up except your feet will be elevated approximately two to three feet. Use a stool, chair, box, or anything available. This will shift more of your body weight to your upper body, making it harder to push up. This is analogous to adding more weight onto the bar when doing a bench press.

Personally, I add these for variation when I do regular pushups.

# Chapter Twelve

## SQUAT

It has been said many times that if you only do one exercise for making the entire body stronger, it should be squats.

Squats engage and contract every major muscle group in the body, as well as getting your heart rate up. This will have the same effect on your cardiovascular system as jogging or sprinting, depending on the intensity.

There are many different types of squats, and all have various levels of intensity. We are only going to focus on 3. These three are all that are needed for strength.

They are called the Hindu, Sumo, and Split squats.

Before we get into the details, here is a short story.

## GAMA THE GREAT

Ghulam Muhammad, known as the "Great" Gama, was India's greatest wrestler. He was 5'9 and weighed about 230 lbs. and was a very strong guy. He was the Indian National Champion in 1909 and retired undefeated after participating in over 5,000 matches.

Why would I mention this guy?

He was famous for his leg workout routine of doing 500 Hindu squats a day to stay in top condition. Nothing was ever mentioned about him lifting weights.

## The Hindu Squat

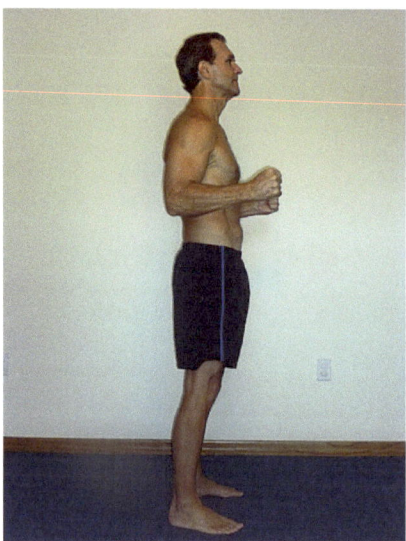

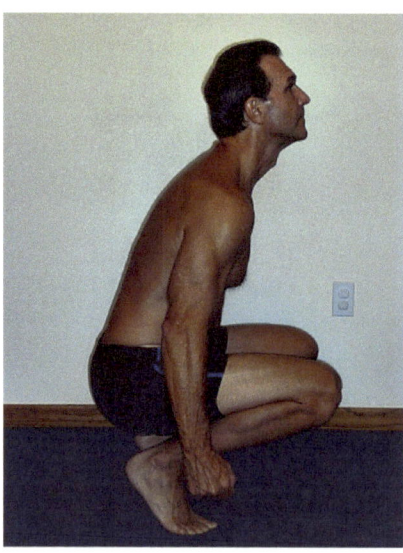

(See illustrations)

This exercise will work your quadriceps (front of the thigh), hamstrings (back of the thigh), calves, abdominals, and lower back.

Hindu squats are said to be the best leg workout that one could possibly do.
This exercise originated in ancient India. They are also known as Tiger squats or Bethaks (Indian name).

Here is how to perform them:

• Start with you feet shoulder-width apart with arms extended out from your chest parallel to the ground.

• Inhale deeply as you clench your fists and pull them towards your chest

• Try to keep your back as straight as possible while lowering your body by bending your knees.

• As you are lowering your body to a tippy-toe position, simultaneously exhaling while extending your arms behind you. Sounds simple, right?

• At the bottom of the exercise you should be up on your toes, keeping your back as straight as possible, with all your breath exhaled completely. Your knuckles or finger tips should lightly be brushing the ground at this time in a continuous motion from behind to in front of you.

• Start to get back to the starting position by pushing off your toes and straightening your legs.

• While you are doing this, simultaneously be inhaling deeply and swing your arms forward in a rowing motion and then back to the starting position with arms at your side, fists clenched, shoulders back, head up, and your lungs filled with air.

Now you are ready to repeat the movement.

## *Important Points:*

• This should be a very smooth, fluid motion. You may vary the speed. DO NOT compromise form for speed. As you get stronger your speed will increase with good form.

• Breathing should always be consistent. The intensity of your inhalations and exhalations will vary depending on your fitness level.

• Always be working at keeping your back as straight as possible at all times.

• When you are in the standing position with your lungs filled with air, arch your back while bringing your chest up and out and your shoulder blades back and down.

• When you perform this movement correctly, your arms should look like you are rowing a boat.

• As with all movements, do not focus on how many repetitions you can do. Focus on perfecting the movement.

Remember, you are not exercising.

**YOU ARE PRACTICING A MOVEMENT TO PERFECTION.**

**The Sumo Squat**

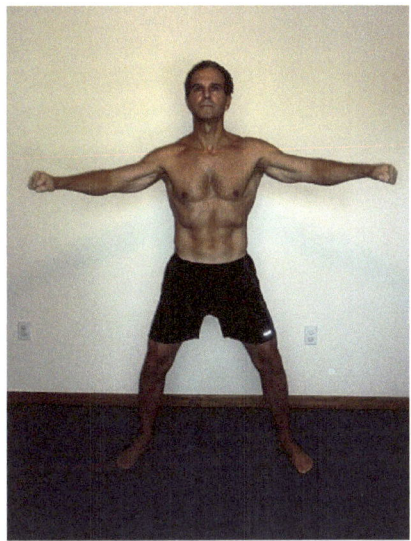

**Squat no lower than parallel to floor**

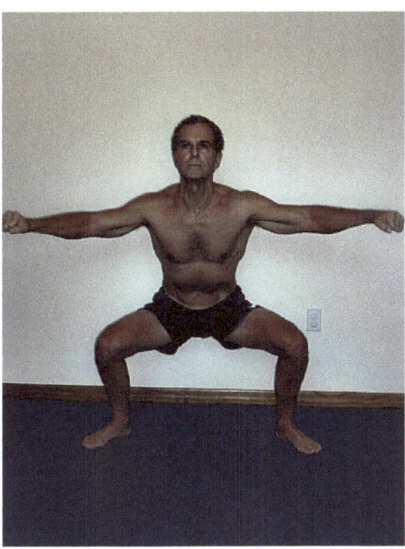

(See illustrations)

This type of squat got its name from the stance of the Sumo wrestlers of Japan. These are very large and strong guys.

I don't quite get it, but Sumo wrestling seems to be a very popular sport in Japan.

The Sumo Squat works basically the same muscles as the Hindu squat, but a lot more emphasis on the glutes (butt).

Here is how to perform them:

• Start with your feet much wider than your hips, just like a Sumo wrestler.

• Point your feet about 45 degrees.

• Arms in front of your body with elbows bent.

• Keep your back straight, chest out and concentrate on keeping your abs tight throughout the movement.

• Lower your body to a comfortable depth or until your thighs are parallel to the floor. This is as deep as you should go without straining your knees. Think about sitting back rather than squatting down. If you cannot get to parallel just go half way or a quarter of the way. In time, with practice, you will be at parallel.

• Breathing is the opposite of the Hindu squat. Inhale while lowering yourself, exhale while rising to a standing position. It is important to do this correctly. Proper breathing creates internal pressure in the abs and chest. This will help to support your spine during the movement.

• At the bottom of the movement push off with your heels while squeezing your glutes and innner thighs until you are back in the starting position.  Keep your back straight the entire movement.

• As with all the movements, focus on the quality, not the amount of repetitions.  Control the tempo (speed) and try not to lose your balance.  Watching yourself in the mirror while performing all the squatting movements will help perfect your form.

**The Split Squat**

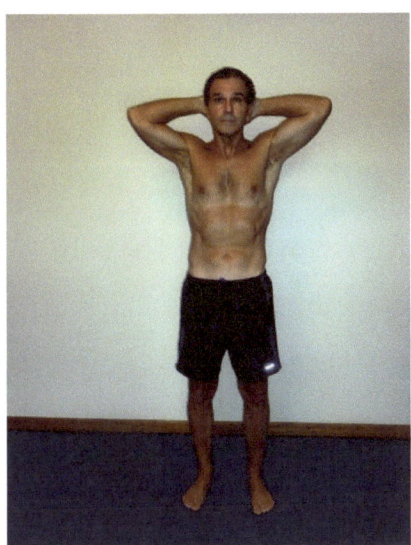

**Keep your head up and back straight**

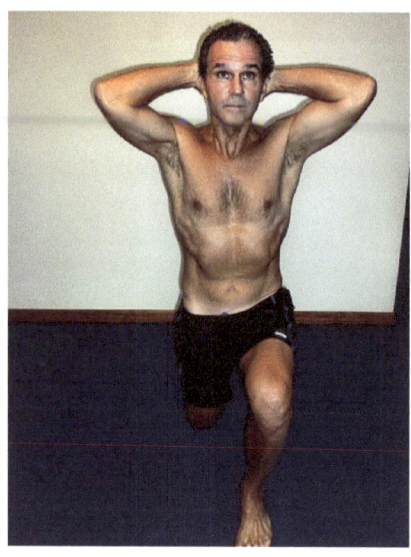

(See illustrations)

This movement is also called the lunge.

There are many possible variations but we will be focusing on the basic movement. The only variation will be the distance that your foot is extended. This will work the same basic muscles as the first two squats, with a little more emphasis on the glutes and hamstrings.

Here is how to perform them:

• Stand up straight with your shoulders back and your hands folded behind your neck. If you prefer, put your arms by your side, but try to get used to the other way.

• Your feet should be hip width apart.

• Keeping your feet hip width apart, take a big step forward with either leg then slowly lower your body into a lunge position. The front knee will bend to a 90 degree angle.

- Make sure the front knee does not move past the tip of the toes. This can put a great deal of strain on the knee joint and cause more harm than good.

- Keep the rear knee bent and the weight up on the ball on the foot. Gently touch your knee on the ground. Remember that your feet should still be hip width apart to help keep you balanced.

- Keep your shoulders back and your torso upright. Keep looking ahead rather than down towards the ground.

- Forcefully push back up to the starting position, pushing from your heel.

- Repeat with same leg or alternate legs, whichever you prefer.

- Do not lean forward at any time during the movement.

## *Important Points:*

- Always remember to keep your abs tight during the entire movement. This will keep your core tight and protect your lower back.

- The bigger your step, the harder the movement, and the more stretch for the hips.

- If you are just starting out, take a smaller step and don't go all the way to the floor with your knee.

- Slowly build up to the full movement.

- Breathe normally throughout the movement.

- Remember, focus on perfection, not repetitions.

# Chapter Thirteen

# PULL

This is the third and final movement.  Like the first two movements, this will have 3 exercises.
All these movements work your back, biceps, forearms, and shoulders.

The first movement is strictly a beginners exercise to condition the muscles to be able to perform
the next two.  Once you can move on, you won't be doing this again.

I call this one The Towel Pull.

(See illustrations)

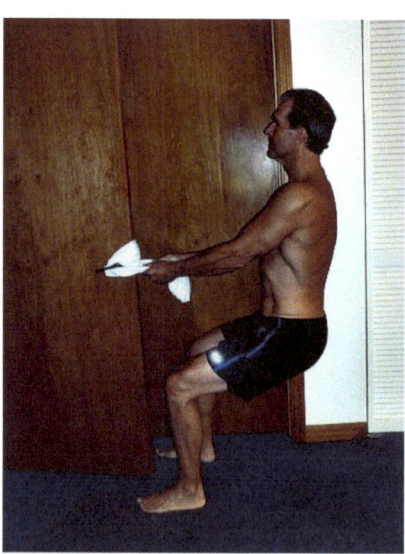

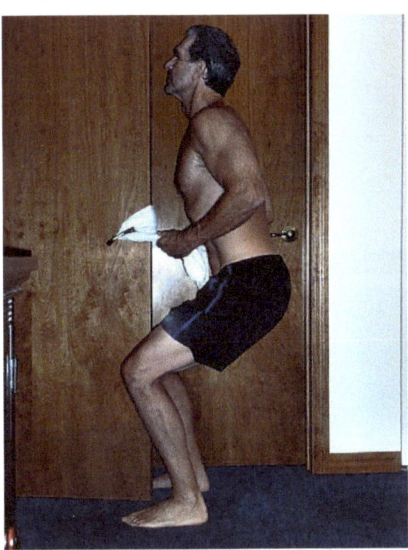

**Move feet forward to make more challenging**

Here is how to perform them:

- Wrap a towel (or t shirt) around the handle of an open door.

- Grab the ends of the towel with both hands.

- Get into a squatting position.

- Pull forward slowly until your chest touches the door.

- Slowly extend your arms until you are back to the starting position.

**Important Points:**

This movement is only for the purpose of getting you strong enough for the next two movements.

Skip this if you are able to do the next two.

Keep this as an alternative if you find yourself in a place without a pull bar, such as a motel room when traveling.

This movement will get more difficult as you move your feet forward.

## The Pull-Up

To do this one and the next, you will need some type of a bar. This is the only piece of equipment needed in the System. A basic door frame bar cost around $20. Very inexpensive investment for the benefits to be gained.

(See illustrations)

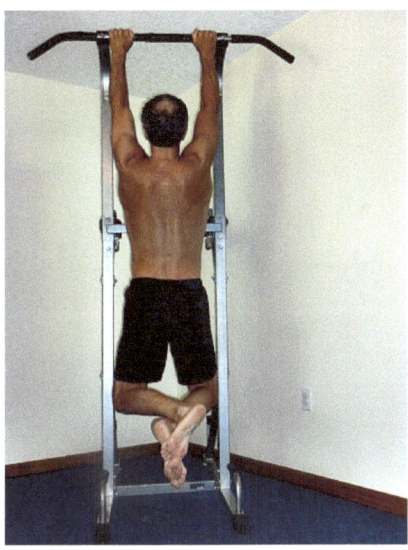

**Just hanging will build your strength**

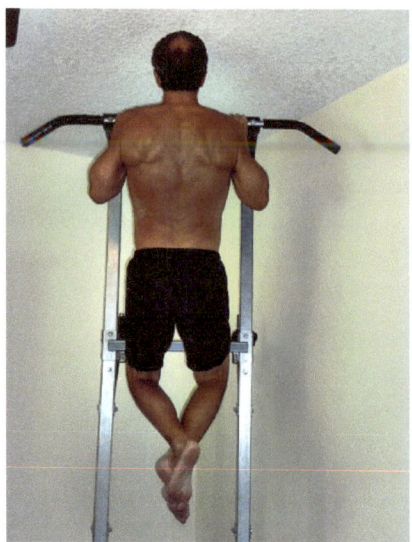

This movement and the next one are the only two that you should warm up before starting. The warm up should first be to just hang by both hands and stretch. Make sure you are using all your weight. You'll find out that hanging alone is fairly strenuous.

If you are unable to perform at least one pull-up, just hanging is another great starting point. Keep trying to increase your hang time, you will get stronger.

After the hanging stretch, then go through the pull up motion about 10 times. This will warm up the muscles used for the actual movement.

Here is how to perform them:

• Grab the bar with a grip slightly wider than shoulder width. Your hands should be in a pronated position, which means facing away from you.

• Hang for a few seconds before beginning.

- Pull yourselves up until your chin is above the bar.

- Keep your body as strait and tensed as possible.

- Slowly lower yourself all the way back down.

Repeat until form is compromised.

## Important Points:

Varying your grip, narrow to wide will work the muscle in a different way.

**Caution:  Don't go too wide or your shoulders could suffer from the strain**.  I know this for a fact.  Go as narrow as you like, even to the point where your hands are touching.

Do not wrap your thumbs around the bar, keep them out of play.

Do not breathe deeply during this movement.  Short, shallow breathes while keeping your abdominals tensed.

## The Chin-Up

(See illustrations)

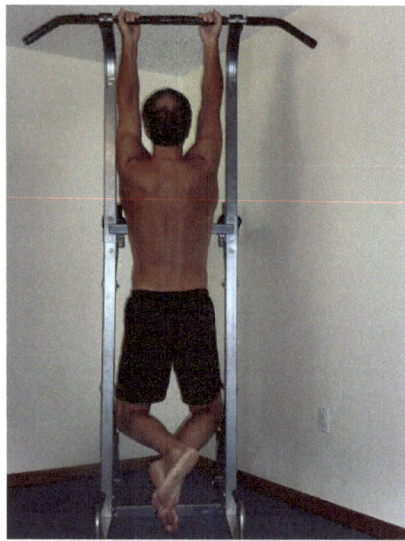

**Your biceps are worked more doing chin ups**

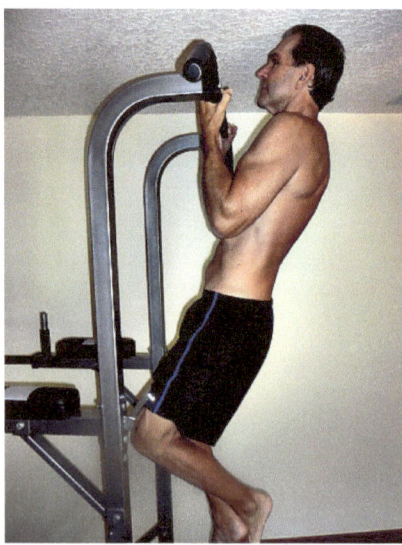

Perform this exactly like the Pull-Up with one exception.

In this movement your hands are supinated. That means your palms are facing you.

This movement works the same body parts as the Pull-Ups with a little more emphasis on your biceps.

## Important Points:

Just hanging from the bar is a good thing to do for stretching and for grip/forearm strength. Remember to tense your core while you hang.

If you cannot do one Pull Up or Chin Up yet, try to get half-way up, or even a quarter of the way. Count these as repetitions for your log. They aren't perfect yet, but they will be soon.

Negatives are another movement to practice if you are not able to do one good repetition. Get your chin over the bar by having someone lift you, or stand on a chair.

Then slowly lower yourself all the way down and let your arms hang for about 5 or 6 seconds. This will get your arms used to supporting your weight.

Breathe very shallow while performing these movements. This will help to keep you tighter.

Remember, you are practicing the movement to perfection. Don't focus on how many repetitions you can get. Focus on how good you can perform each repetition.

# Chapter Fourteen


# Putting It All Together


Now that you've seen all the parts of the System, let's put them all together in a simple workable way.

First, decide when you are going to start. Hopefully you will start today rather than tomorrow.

Try to incorporate the System into one of your daily routines. For instance, I do mine in the mornings in between getting my Boys ready for school and getting myself ready for the day.

You may find the afternoon or evening works best for your schedule. You may even find that sometimes a few minutes in the morning and a few in the evening works better on some days. It all counts.

Next, try to get your picture taken. Either by yourself through a mirror or have someone take it. Then date it and file it away for 3 to 4 months. This will be extremely motivating when you compare the pictures in a few months.

Next, make sure you have several Weekly Log sheets (see Resources section) printed. Fill in the dates for the first week.

Don't forget a simple tape measure.

Now you're ready to practice the movements and record every Push, Squat, and Pull repetition you do for each day.

If you are just getting started trying to get back in shape, I would recommend doing one movement from the Push, Squat, and Pull every day, six days a week, for about 4 weeks. If you can eventually do two or three sets of each, great.

If you are in good condition, you could concentrate on Push movements one day, Squat movements the second day, and Pull movements the third day. Then start again with Push movements the fourth day, Squat the fifth day, and Pull the sixth day, rest on day seven.

This way you are able to do multiple sets (of three different movements) all working the same muscle groups. In the example above, you would be working your entire body completely, twice a week.

Personally I like doing the Pull and Push movements three days a week (every other day). Then I do Squats on the alternate days. This way I work every muscle group three times a week. I do mix it up on occasion.

Find a starting point that works for you and just start.

If you have questions you have support on www.6PackAfter60.com.

# Chapter Fifteen

# The Spill-Over Effect

After you have been faithfully using this system for a few months, at least four to six, you will start to experience the spill-over effect. I need to emphasize that key word "faithfully". Faithfully means at least five days a week and hopefully six.

What is the spill-over effect?

Because you have disciplined yourself and have started to reap the benefits, you'll notice other improvements in your life.

Possible spill-over examples:

• You may have lost weight. Because of the consistent physical activity you are burning more calories than you are taking in. The more intense the movements the more calories you burn. Your intensity will increase with time.

• You may have lost weight because your are more conscious of the food choices you make. If this is you, you've learned that you don't need to be on a diet to lose weight. You just need to make better choices.

• You may have more confidence because you are getting stronger and more in control of how you look and feel.

- You may find that you are getting along better with people. This could happen because you are feeling happier and more relaxed. Physical activity, especially the strenuous kind, stimulates various brain chemicals that make this happen.

- You may find yourself getting more organized.

- Your concentration may increase because you have been practicing focus during all the movements.

- You will definitely have more energy and stamina so you may find yourself doing more things than you used to do and doing things longer than you used to do them.

- You might find that you are able to fall asleep faster and deepen your sleep. Make sure you don't exercise too close to bedtime. Exercise has an energizing affect which could make it hard to sleep.

- You might start getting more ideas and start more projects.

I could go on, but you see my point. There are numerous benefits to staying with the System.

In conclusion, I wish you much success with this new venture.

I would love to hear all your stories.

Please write to me at Jim@6PackAfter60.com

# Resources

## Weekly PSP System Log

| Date | Day | Movement | Set 1 | Set 2 | Set 3 | Movement | Set 1 | Set 2 | Set 3 | Movement | Set 1 | Set 2 | Set 3 |
|------|-----|----------|-------|-------|-------|----------|-------|-------|-------|----------|-------|-------|-------|
|  | Mon | Push |  |  |  | Squat |  |  |  | Pull |  |  |  |
|  | Tues | Push |  |  |  | Squat |  |  |  | Pull |  |  |  |
|  | Wed | Push |  |  |  | Squat |  |  |  | Pull |  |  |  |
|  | Thurs | Push |  |  |  | Squat |  |  |  | Pull |  |  |  |
|  | Fri | Push |  |  |  | Squat |  |  |  | Pull |  |  |  |
|  | Sat | Push |  |  |  | Squat |  |  |  | Pull |  |  |  |
|  | Sun | Push |  |  |  | Squat |  |  |  | Pull |  |  |  |

**Totals:**
*(for the week)*

| | |
|---|---|
| Push: |  |
| Squat: |  |
| Pull: |  |

Weight: [ ]
Waist: [ ]

## Monthly PSP System Log

| | Jan | Feb | March | April | May | June | July | Aug | Sept | Oct | Nov | Dec | Total |
|---|---|---|---|---|---|---|---|---|---|---|---|---|---|
| Push-Ups | | | | | | | | | | | | | |
| Squats | | | | | | | | | | | | | |
| Pull-ups | | | | | | | | | | | | | |
| Beginning Weight: | | | | | | | | | | | | | |
| Ending Weight: | | | | | | | | | | | | | |